better **nutrition** *magazine* presents

CH00952056

CHOLESTEROL

by **MATTHEW BUDOFF, MD, FACC, FAHA**

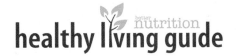

healthy living guide

Published by:
Active Interest Media, Inc.
300 N. Continental Blvd., Suite 650
El Segundo, CA 90245

This booklet is part of the *Better Nutrition Healthy Living Guide* series. For more information, visit www.betternutrition.com. Better Nutrition magazine is available at fine natural health stores throughout the United States. Design by Aline Design: Bellingham, Wash.

The information in this booklet is for educational purposes only and is not recommended as a means of diagnosing or treating an illness. All health matters should be supervised by a qualified healthcare professional. The publisher and the author(s) are not responsible for individuals who choose to self-diagnose and/or self-treat.

CHOLESTEROL

CONTENTS

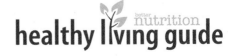

Introduction
Keep The Beat

When functioning properly, the human heart beats more than 100,000 times and pumps about 2,000 gallons of blood through your vessels every day. Millions of sophisticated heart cells intricately orchestrate the continual pumping of blood and oxygen through your veins. Your heart is about the size of your hand, and all of your arteries and blood vessels, if laid end-to-end, would circle the earth twice.

The beating of the heart keeps oxygen and nutrient-rich blood flowing throughout the body. The heart circulates blood and oxygen out to the body's tissues and organs and then circulates it back to the lungs where it can be reoxygenated. After the lungs reoxygenate the blood, some of the blood is filtered through the kidneys and liver. The kidneys cleanse the blood of waste products and then eliminate the waste via urine. The heart is divided into two sides. One side pumps "fresh," oxygenated blood out to the body, and the other side receives the oxygen-deficient blood. While the heart fills up with oxygen-deficient blood, it is considered "at rest." The heart contracts as it pushes the oxygenated blood out.

Road Block

The seemingly simple operation of the heart is rife with risks that can damage our health and cause death. The single most dangerous outcome to the heart and your health is the blockage of an artery. The most common form of heart disease is known as coronary artery disease, which simply means that blood flow through the arteries has become blocked or obstructed. This reduces blood flow to the heart and can cause other heart problems such as angina (chest pain) and myocardial infarction (heart attack).

Your arteries start out flexible and elastic. Over time, the arteries can become thick, stiff, and susceptible to plaque buildup. This is known as atherosclerosis or hardening of the arteries. No one is born with hardening of the arteries. It is caused by a gradual, silent buildup of plaque that can eventually be deadly.

Plaque is a combination of substances including fat and cholesterol. Without plaque, blood can flow freely as the heart maintains its healthy beating. When plaque builds up, the artery narrows, constricting blood flow to the heart. Plaque can even build up to the point where blood flow is completely blocked. When there is too much cholesterol in the body,

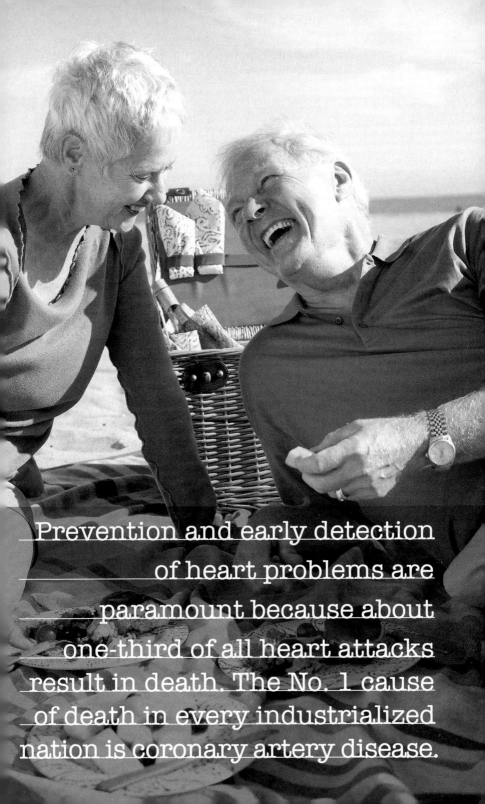

Prevention and early detection of heart problems are paramount because about one-third of all heart attacks result in death. The No. 1 cause of death in every industrialized nation is coronary artery disease.

plaque can accumulate. High cholesterol is a risk factor for the development of heart disease. Other risk factors include:

- High blood pressure
- High homocysteine levels
- Smoking
- Obesity
- Diabetes
- Inactivity
- Increased and uncontrolled stress and anxiety
- Poor diet

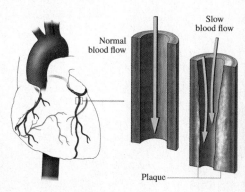

The next chapter will review diet and lifestyle factors associated with high cholesterol. While it is not the only risk factor for developing heart disease, high cholesterol remains a key concern for many Americans. There is no question that elevated cholesterol can disrupt the rhythmic beating of the heart. Researchers have discovered, however, that it is the combination of elevated cholesterol with high homocysteine levels that presents an increased risk for heart problems.

Oxidation And Your Heart

According to groundbreaking researcher Kilmer McCully, MD, high cholesterol levels alone do not cause heart disease. "When it [cholesterol] is taken up into the arterial wall, it becomes oxidized or modified, and it has damaging effects on cells in the arterial wall," says McCully. Homocysteine is one reason why cholesterol may build up in the artery to dangerous levels.

Homocysteine is a nonessential amino acid that results from a deficiency of three B vitamins: B6, B12, and folic acid. In addition, too much dietary protein and too little of these B vitamins can convert methionine, an essential amino acid, into its toxic byproduct, homocysteine. Some researchers believe high homocysteine poses a greater risk for heart disease than high blood pressure, smoking, or high cholesterol.

As researchers dig deeper into the issue of elevated homocysteine, they are finding that the health ramifications of this condition are broad. It could, in fact, be the catalyst cholesterol needs to begin blocking the artery. Both homocysteine and cholesterol levels should be considered when creating a health plan. But before we can construct that plan, we need to first understand what cholesterol is and why it is so important to keep levels in a healthy range.

Chapter One
Understanding Cholesterol

High cholesterol is a risk factor for heart disease. A risk factor is a habit, trait, or condition that increases your risk of having a heart attack. There are two types of risk factors: those that can be modified and those that can't. Risk factors that cannot be modified are gender, family history, and age. High cholesterol is a modifiable risk factor. In other words, by using a proactive approach, you can reverse it.

Well over 100 million Americans—about 17 percent of the population—have moderate to high cholesterol levels. Of these, more than 37 million have cholesterol levels that place them at high risk of developing heart disease. But the fact remains, not all cholesterol is bad.

Your body needs cholesterol. It is manufactured primarily in the liver from fragments of proteins, fats, and carbohydrates. Cholesterol is absolutely critical to the:

- Production of vitamin D, an important nutrient that helps prevent many illnesses
- Formation of sex hormones such as estrogen, testosterone, and progesterone
- Production of bile acids that help us digest food
- Formation and maintenance of various cell membranes, specifically in the brain and central nervous system.

If cholesterol is so important, then why is it considered so dangerous? Because when there is too much, it can encourage plaque buildup. The body makes as much cholesterol as needed. Unfortunately, cholesterol has become a key "ingredient" of the typical American diet. In addition, medications, genetics, lack of exercise, and many other factors can cause an individual to have too much cholesterol. The first step to controlling cholesterol is to test cholesterol levels.

Diagnosis

Having high cholesterol will not produce symptoms. Therefore, the only way to determine if you have high cholesterol is by having your doctor check your cholesterol levels. It is absolutely critical to properly detect and diagnose high cholesterol. Current guidelines from the American Heart Association (AHA) and others recommend that everyone have a baseline cholesterol test before age 20 and then every five years thereafter.

One of the most common ways to determine cholesterol levels is with a simple blood test. The test measures cholesterol and triglycerides that are circulating in your blood. Triglycerides are a type of fat in the blood. Similar to cholesterol, if triglycerides become elevated, you may be at an increased risk of heart disease. To get the most accurate cholesterol test result, do not eat or drink anything for nine to 12 hours prior to the blood test. This includes beverages such as coffee, tea, or soda. Only drink water.

However, some patients with high cholesterol never develop heart disease, while others have normal cholesterol levels and have heart attacks early in life. It has been recognized that the only accurate way to gauge your level of plaque build-up is a test called a heart scan. This CAT scan allows direct visualization of the coronary arteries and detects plaque years or decades before the buildup becomes severe enough to cause a heart attack or blockages that require surgery or stents to open. This CAT scan, also known as a calcium scan or cardiac CT, only exposes the person to a small radiation dose (the equivalent of a woman getting a mammogram or a child getting dental X-rays) and does not require needles, injections, or dye. This scan has been shown to detect risk of heart disease better than carotid tests, C-reactive protein (a measure of inflammation in the blood) and exercise tests (treadmill or nuclear testing). This noninvasive test is poised to change the way we look at adults' risk for heart disease and is recommended by the AHA and American College of Cardiology, along with the National Cholesterol Education Panel, as a preeminent method to detect patients at increased risk of heart attacks in the next few years. For more information about this test, visit www.calciumscan.com or call (310) 222-2773.

Medical Therapy

Keep in mind that some drugs can either increase or decrease your total cholesterol levels. Be sure to inform your doctor of all drugs and/or dietary supplements you may be taking. Some drugs can interfere with cholesterol test results. These include:

- Anabolic steroids
- Beta blockers
- Corticosteroids
- Birth control pills
- Sulfanomides
- MAO inhibitors
- Statins

The blood cholesterol test measures both low-density lipoprotein (LDL) cholesterol and high-density lipoprotein (HDL) cholesterol. The reason both types are important is because only LDL cholesterol is bad. HDL cholesterol is considered "good" because it transports excess cholesterol to the liver for metabolism and elimination from the body. The reason LDL cholesterol is considered bad is because it sticks more easily to the arterial wall and can build up as plaque.

Your total cholesterol should be less than 200 mg/dl, and your LDL should be less than 130 mg/dl. Your HDL should be greater than 40 mg/dl. You have high cholesterol if your total cholesterol is 240 mg/dl or higher. An LDL of more than 160 mg/dl and an HDL below 40 mg/dl are considered high risk. For more information, refer to the chart on this page. Newer data suggests that lower targets (LDL less than 100 mg/dl) may be more appropriate for people who have either suffered a heart attack or are at very high risk of experiencing heart problems.

CHOLESTEROL MEASUREMENT

Total Cholesterol	LDL	HDL
Desirable = below 200 mg/dl	below 100 mg/dl	60 mg/dl and above
Borderline high risk = 200 to 239 mg/dl	130 to 159 mg/dl	40 to 59 mg/dl
High risk = 240 mg/dl	160 mg/dl or higher	below 40 mg/dl

Testing for inflammation is thought to be helpful in identifying risk. However, this type of testing (i.e., C-reactive protein or CRP testing) has not been shown to be a reliable predictor because anything can elevate inflammation levels, including infections, arthritis, and cancer. Thus, elevations of these proteins are more often not related to heart disease and are not useful as measures of risk or to track progression of heart disease.

Conventional Treatment

If your cholesterol is high, your doctor may recommend a cholesterol-lowering prescription drug. These drugs are known as statins, and they are currently the only FDA-approved prescription drugs for reducing LDL cholesterol. Some of the most popular brands of statin drugs include Lipitor, Crestor, Zocor, and Mevacor. Statins can be effective in certain cases because they block a substance that the body needs to make cholesterol. Some of these drugs may also help your body reabsorb accumulated cholesterol to help prevent plaque buildup.

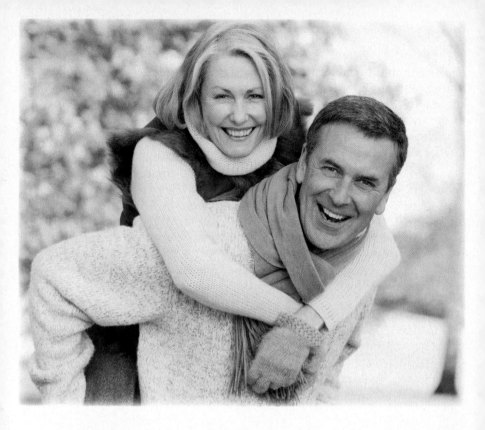

Because these drugs have side effects, before considering taking a statin, ask yourself these two questions:

What are all your risk factors for heart disease in addition to high cholesterol?

What exactly are the side effects of the prescription being recommended?

Remember, high cholesterol is just one factor that puts you at risk of developing heart disease or having a heart attack. If high cholesterol is your only risk factor, you may want to try other means to lower your cholesterol before taking a prescription medication. Chapters Three and Four provide information about a natural approach to keeping cholesterol levels in check. If you have a healthy diet, are physically active, and have tried dietary supplements, then a statin drug may be indicated in some cases. Unless they don't tolerate these drugs, some patients need to be on statins. These include people with diabetes, those with known coronary disease (including heart attack, stroke, or bypass surgery), and individuals with very high risk of having a heart attack (such as those with a positive heart scan). In clinical studies, statin drugs have been shown to reduce the risk of all-cause death (improved survival) when taken by patients at high risk. The American Diabetes Association recommends statins for all diabetic persons over the age of 40. Also, almost everyone who is at risk for heart disease should be taking a low dose (81 mg per day) of aspirin, as this has also been shown to lower cardiovascular risk by about one-third. This means that the combination of aspirin and a statin reduces chances of heart attack, stroke, and cardiac death by over 50 percent.

Discuss all of your options with your doctor. If you are already taking a statin, do not discontinue taking it without first consulting with your doctor. You should never discontinue taking any prescription medication without your doctor's knowledge.

Weigh the decision to take a statin very carefully because taking a statin drug is most likely a lifelong commitment. Even if your cholesterol comes down, you'll likely have to stay on your statin medication indefinitely because there is a good chance your cholesterol will go back up once you discontinue the medication. In some cases, making significant diet and lifestyle changes may help you discontinue your medication completely. But again, you need to discuss these options with your doctor. The side effects of statin drugs include:

- Muscle and joint aches and pains
- Liver damage
- Nausea
- Diarrhea
- Constipation
- Deficiency of coenzyme Q10 (CoQ10)

Depletion of CoQ10 is concerning because CoQ10 is so important to optimal heart function. For individuals who are taking statins, I recommend a minimum dosage of 60 mg of CoQ10 daily. I recommend a product called Kyolic Formula 110 because it combines CoQ10 with aged garlic extract. I'll provide more information about aged garlic extract and CoQ10 in Chapter Three.

Perhaps the most concerning side effects of statins are liver and kidney damage. These drugs can cause an increase in liver enzymes, so a liver test should be done periodically while statins are being used. Increased liver enzymes can lead to permanent liver damage. In some cases, statins cause muscle cells to break down and release a protein that can damage the kidneys. Taking certain drugs and drinking alcohol in excess can magnify these side effects.

Statin drugs have become big business. In 2007, according to CBS News, the most commonly prescribed cholesterol-lowering drug, Lipitor, had annual sales in excess of $12 billion. While these drugs have saved many lives, such widespread use may not be necessary. A targeted approach that employs statins for certain individuals—such as those with atherosclerosis on a calcium scan, diabetes, or known heart disease—is the best way to use these drugs.

The most effective natural approach to lowering cholesterol and keeping homocysteine levels in check begins with diet and lifestyle.

As for homocysteine drugs, the FDA has approved betaine (brand name Cystadane) for lowering homocysteine levels. In addition to Cystadane, doctors often also recommend taking a dietary supplement that contains vitamins B6, B12, and folic acid (also known as folate). According to the National Institutes of Health (NIH), betaine has side effects, some serious, including:

- Nausea
- Diarrhea
- Vomiting
- Headache
- Drowsiness
- Confusion
- Behavior changes
- Seizures
- Loss of consciousness

If you are taking this drug, tell your doctor if you experience any of the previously listed side effects. Also, if you are pregnant or plan on becoming pregnant, you should avoid Cystadane.

The most effective natural approach to lowering cholesterol and keeping homocysteine levels in check begins with diet and lifestyle. Many prestigious medical journals, including the *Journal of the American Medical Association* (JAMA), report that drug therapy should be recommended only after dietary modifications have been proven unsuccessful and high risk factors are not present.

Chapter Two
Diet And Lifestyle

We've all heard the saying "You are what you eat." It makes sense then that if you eat a high cholesterol diet, you will have high cholesterol. As mentioned previously, the body manufactures the cholesterol it needs. To function properly, the body requires the vitamins, minerals, amino acids, and other nutrients it gleans from food. Although cholesterol is important, the body does not need any more than it can make. That's why paying attention to the cholesterol content of your food becomes critical if you are to control or reduce cholesterol.

Less of These

The United States government has established a Recommended Dietary Allowance (RDA) for key nutrients our body needs to function properly. There is no RDA for cholesterol, but there is a maximum recommended daily dosage. While a diet that provides very little cholesterol is optimal, the AHA recommends we keep our total daily cholesterol to 300 mg or less. If for breakfast you have a glass of whole milk, an egg, and a piece of toast with butter, you have reached the AHA recommendation of cholesterol for the entire day. For a list of cholesterol amounts for some common foods, refer to the sidebar "Cholesterol Content of Some Common Foods" on page 14.

From a practical standpoint, it's important to read product labels. Reading food labels is a good habit to get into for a number of reasons including finding out the cholesterol content of the foods you are eating. The cholesterol amount will nearly always be listed on the products you choose. Remember, just because something says, "lean" or "low-fat" does not mean it is low in cholesterol.

Most dairy based foods are high in cholesterol.

Some foods don't have labels or listed cholesterol amounts. It's important to be aware of foods that can sabotage your cholesterol-lowering efforts. Limit your intake of common high cholesterol foods including:

- Eggs
- Whole milk
- Butter
- Cream, cream cheese, and ice cream
- Shellfish such as shrimp
- Organ meats such as kidney or liver
- Duck and goose

As you can see, high cholesterol foods are primarily animal products. By reducing the amount of animal products you eat, you will reduce the amount of cholesterol in your diet. One of the goals of a healthy cholesterol program is to increase levels of HDL, the good cholesterol. Keep in mind, however, that there are no food sources of this good cholesterol. All dietary sources of cholesterol can become dangerous when eaten in excess, especially for individuals who have already been diagnosed with high cholesterol or those who have a family history of high cholesterol.

A great diet that I often recommend is the *South Beach Diet*, created by my colleague and friend Arthur Agatston, MD. The book *The South Beach Diet* discusses in detail the issues of "white foods," including white rice, white bread, potatoes, and pasta. These calories (based in carbohydrates) come with virtually no redeeming qualities and don't fill us up, so we keep eating. Remember the last time you went to an Italian restaurant and

Cholesterol Content of Some Common Foods

FOOD	mg
Liver (3 oz pan-fried)	324
Egg (extra large)	245
Shrimp (6-8 breaded and fried)	200
Duck (1/2, roasted meat only)	197
Cheese (1 cup whole-milk ricotta)	125
Milk (1 cup whole)	35
Sour Cream (2 Tbsp)	20

Source: United States Department of Agriculture

had a whole bowl of warm bread and then continued to eat a full meal. Or think of your experiences at Mexican restaurants with the bowls of chips and salsa they serve. These white foods provide a lot of calories yet fail to fill us up, so we keep eating. Fortunately, there are some great-tasting foods that we should keep eating if we want to control cholesterol.

More of These

It's not surprising that fruits, vegetables, and grains do not contain any cholesterol. This is still another reason why increasing your consumption of these foods is critical to your health. And if you need one more reason to increase your daily intake of fruits and vegetables, do it because they contain valuable B vitamins.

To keep homocysteine levels in check, we need to get enough of three key B vitamins via our diet and dietary supplements. Healthy food sources for these key B vitamins include:

- Vitamin B6 = seeds, beans, bananas, fortified oatmeal, spinach, and avocado
- Vitamin B12 = fish and fortified cereals
- Folic Acid = green leafy vegetables, citrus fruits, fortified grains, beans, and peas

In 2007 the FDA reviewed the scientific literature on five specific foods proven to be beneficial to the heart. As a result of that review, the FDA has decided to give these foods a health claim for managing cholesterol. In addition to vegetables and fruits, individuals wishing to lower their cholesterol should increase their daily intake of the following five cholesterol-lowering foods:

- Fatty fish (e.g. salmon, trout, tuna)
- Oatmeal
- Oat bran
- Walnuts
- Foods fortified with plant sterols (more about plant sterols in Chapter Three)

Some studies have shown that a vegetarian diet that includes fish can help lower cholesterol levels. Several European studies have demonstrated that vegetarians have fewer risk factors for cardiovascular disease, including high cholesterol. A recent study published in *The Chinese Journal of Physiology* showed that postmenopausal vegetarian women had lower LDL cholesterol and triglyceride levels. In addition to eliminating animal products, vegetarians typically also have a higher intake of whole grains, oatmeal, oat bran, nuts, beans, fruits, and vegetables, which can also help explain why they have lower cholesterol levels.

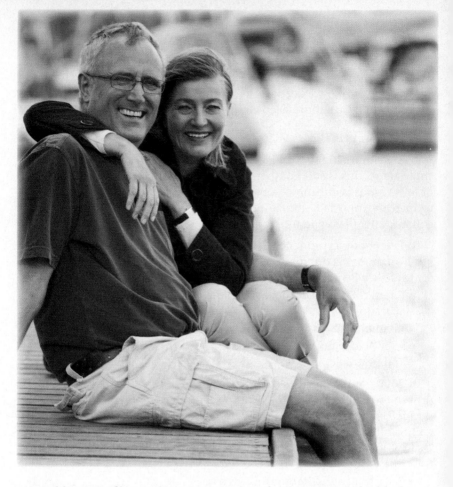

In addition to fiber and B vitamins, plant foods contain valuable, heart-healthy compounds called sterols. These compounds have been shown to reduce cholesterol. For more information about plant sterols, refer to Chapter Three.

Good Fats

Another problem with animal foods is that they are high in saturated fat. A quick lesson in fats tells us that there are good fats and bad fats. Saturated fats are bad fats that can weaken the immune system and clog arteries. Trans fats are synthetically created liquid fats and are also considered very bad fats. Trans fats are so dangerous that in January 2006, all food manufacturers were required to list the amounts of both saturated and trans fats on the label. Prior to this, consumers did not know how much trans fats were in the foods they were eating. Some states have even banned trans fats from being used in restaurants.

An Ideal Cholesterol-Lowering Breakfast

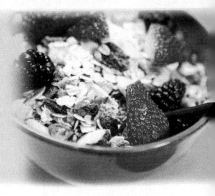

Serves 1

Boil 1 cup water.

Add 1/2 cup organic oats.

Cook on medium heat for 5 minutes.

Add organic, low-fat milk.

Top with walnuts and fresh fruit.

Saturated and trans fats have been clearly linked to a weakened immune system and heart disease. For this reason, all fats have inadvertently been lumped into the same category: bad foods that should be avoided. But the fact is, there are some fats that are absolutely critical to our health and the efficient function of our heart. These fats are called essential fatty acids (EFAs). Two important EFAs are eicosapentaenoic acid (EPA) and docosahexaenoic acid (DHA).

One of the reasons I tell my patients to eat more fish is because they contain EPA and DHA, which have been proven to be beneficial to heart function. These fish oils have been shown in clinical studies to enhance heart health and prevent heart disease. Olive and flax oils are also considered healthy oils. When cooking, avoid vegetable and flax oils because they are susceptible to damage from the heat and can become more toxic to your health. I recommend olive oil for cooking. If you do not eat fish several times a week, you may want to consider supplementing your diet with a quality fish oil supplement. The brand I recommend is Kyolic EPA.

Essential fatty acids, along with the dietary recommendations in this chapter, will also help control inflammation. I agree with the many researchers who feel that inflammation, along with high cholesterol and elevated homocysteine, is a significant contributor to arterial damage and heart disease. An overactive inflammatory response in the arteries can lead to plaque fragments and clots. The foods we eat and the dietary supplements we take on a daily basis can help normalize inflammation, cholesterol, and homocysteine. For this reason, EPA and DHA are important additions to a heart-healthy diet.

Don't Diet

Having a healthy diet will help you maintain a healthy body weight. The research has consistently and conclusively proven that being overweight increases your risk of high cholesterol and heart disease. An interesting fact about weight gain and heart disease involves your waistline. Research indicates that a waist size of less than 40 inches for men and less

Try Kale Chips Instead of Potato Chips

Potato chips are not good for your heart because they are high in fat and sodium and virtually devoid of nutrients. They are the epitome of empty-calorie foods.

Kale is a good source of B vitamins and other nutrients. And if baked properly, they can become a healthful alternative to potato chips. To help you get more kale in your diet, try kale chips. They are a tasty, healthy snack that even kids will appreciate.

1. Separate kale leaves from the stem, and cut or tear them into small, chip-like pieces.
2. Coat with olive oil, and put on a baking sheet.
3. Lightly salt with sea salt (don't use too much salt).
4. Bake at 350°F for 8 to 12 minutes (depending on how crispy you like your chips).

Enjoy!

than 35 inches for women lowers cardiac risk. Focus on making your waist smaller than your hips.

Some people turn to diet pills and nutritional supplements containing ephedra and other stimulants. You should avoid these diet pills and supplements, especially if you have high blood pressure or a family history of heart disease.

In addition to eating at least five servings of fruits and vegetables daily, I recommend the following:

- Eat 20 to 30 grams of fiber each day.
- Drink at least eight 8-ounce glasses of pure water each day (avoid unfiltered tap water).
- Reduce or eliminate simple sugars.
- Alcohol raises your good cholesterol, but strictly limit it to one to two servings per day maximum (for example, a glass of wine, bottle of beer, or shot of hard liquor).
- Choose organic, fresh, unprocessed foods whenever possible, and avoid preservatives, additives, and food colorings.
- Reduce "white foods" including white rice, white bread, potato products, and pastas.
- Reduce sodium and saturated fat intake.

Avoid the temptation of jumping on the next diet bandwagon. Healthy, long-lasting weight loss requires dietary adjustments that you can live with for a lifetime. When you combine a healthy diet with consistent physical activity, you are well on your way to naturally controlling cholesterol while helping to prevent the No. 1 disease killer of our time—heart disease. Remember, your day-to-day diet and lifestyle choices have a colossal effect on your long-term heart health. Keep everything in moderation so you can enjoy a longer and more enjoyable life.

Keep Moving

Next to diet, physical activity is the most important thing you can do for your heart. Many studies have shown that exercise increases HDL and decreases LDL cholesterol. Exercise also helps reduce body fat, uses up excess sugar in the bloodstream, lowers blood pressure, and trains the heart to pump more efficiently. It also staves off the onset of diabetes. These are all key heart-healthy benefits.

Before you begin a new exercise program, consult with your physician, especially if you have a history of heart disease or high blood pressure and you have been fairly inactive.

In addition to the amazing cardiovascular benefits of exercise, studies have shown that exercise can:

- Stimulate a positive immune response
- Release "feel-good" endorphins in the brain
- Increase oxygen and blood flow to the brain
- Increase bone density and muscle mass

For these reasons, exercise will not only help you prevent heart disease, but it can also help with depression, anxiety, osteoporosis, fatigue, diabetes, and weight loss. Exercise has also been shown to relieve pain, increase

An Ideal After-Dinner or Afternoon Snack

Serves 1

1 cup of bran-based cereal

Add organic, low-fat milk.

Top with raisins and/or bananas.

This type of simple snack provides bran (good for cholesterol and dietary fiber), raisins (good for bowels), and fruit (raisins/bananas).

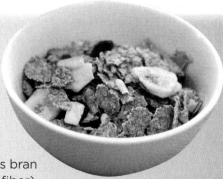

mental sharpness, and improve sleep quality. In general, exercise will help you live longer. There is no pill or surgical procedure available today that can do all that!

Being physically active on a consistent basis is the most important factor. That doesn't necessarily mean going to the gym or participating in formal exercise classes. Some people may prefer gardening, walking, riding the bike, or playing golf several times a week. Be sure to vary your physical activity so you don't get bored or give up. When it comes to exercise, you want to focus on three key areas:

- Aerobic activity (brisk walking, biking, swimming)
- Stretching (yoga, tai chi)
- Strength training (Pilates, weight lifting)

Five Servings: It's Easier Than You Think!

Some of my patients have told me that it seems difficult to consume five servings of fruits and vegetables every day. After you realize that a serving is not really that much, you'll find that five servings isn't overwhelming at all. Each of these is one serving:

- 1 cup of leafy greens or four leaves of lettuce
- $1/2$ cup of raw vegetables
- $1/2$ cup of dried fruit
- 1 medium apple (the size of a tennis ball)

If you create a salad with the above items, you've already eaten four servings, and that's just one meal! While I'm not an advocate of fast-food restaurants in general, you can get a grilled chicken salad with a side of apple slices and cover two servings while increasing your fiber and healthy food intake. If you snack on carrots or celery, you obtain another quick vegetable serving while LOSING WEIGHT (it takes more energy to eat the carrots or celery than you get from the actual vegetables, unless you dip them in fattening salad dressing).

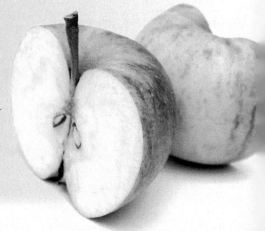

Exercise is one of the most important healthy lifestyle activities you can choose. Here are some exercise tips to keep in mind:

- Make physical activity part of your daily routine.
- An organized exercise routine should include a minimum of 30 minutes, four times a week.
- Choose activities you enjoy, and mix it up to make it fun.
- Be sure to warm up and cool down with simple stretching.
- Make a habit to take the stairs instead of the elevator when feasible.

When you are physically active, you look and feel better. Exercise has been shown to help prevent and even reverse high cholesterol levels. Make exercise a part of your daily heart-healthy plan.

Low-Cholesterol Living

In addition to diet and exercise, there are many proactive things you can do to enhance your heart health and lower your cholesterol. The top two culprits that can sabotage your cholesterol-lowering efforts are smoking and stress.

If you smoke, you need to quit. I know it's not easy, but tobacco use (cigarettes, cigars, snuff) is the single most dangerous lifestyle activity you can choose. Smoking causes heart disease and can trigger a heart attack. The good news is that the benefits of quitting smoking are almost immediate. According to the World Health Organization, just one year after quitting, a previous smoker's risk of heart disease decreases by 50 percent. After 15 years, the risk of dying from heart disease for an ex-smoker is almost identical to someone who has never smoked.

While quitting smoking is the most important thing you will ever do, it may also be one of the most difficult things you do. Here are some things to try:

- Acupuncture = although there are no clinical studies proving the effectiveness of acupuncture to help someone stop smoking, there are many testimonials.
- Cold turkey = if you can make it through the first two weeks, you have a great chance of succeeding.
- Exercise = this will help calm your anxiety and channel your energy away from smoking.
- Hypnotherapy = there are no clinical studies regarding smoking, but clearly many people have benefited from this therapy.
- Props = try chewing gum, holding a cigarette without lighting it, or chewing on carrots or celery.
- Support = surround yourself with people who support your decision to quit.

- Dietary supplements = the herb lobelia has been shown to help some people stop smoking.
- Prescriptions = pills, gum, and even prescription nasal spray can help some smokers quit gradually (be sure to discuss these options thoroughly with your doctor because some have side effects).

Many people say they smoke because it helps calm their nerves. Stress is a big part of our lives. Living with stress and finding healthy ways to cope with it is absolutely critical to controlling cholesterol and preventing heart disease.

In addition to exercise, I recommend finding stress-reduction techniques that you can relate to and incorporate into your daily life. Some healthy relaxation methods include:

- Meditation
- Aromatherapy
- Music
- Journaling
- Being in nature or around animals
- Doing volunteer work
- Talking to supportive friends, family, or a therapist

When we are under stress, it can be tempting to participate in unhealthy behaviors. During times of high stress, try to avoid alcohol, overeating, caffeine, and excessive behaviors like overworking. Do not isolate yourself. Find ways to manage your stress in healthy ways so your body can rebound and rebuild.

Top 10 Tips

Many well-designed clinical studies have clearly shown that there is a connection between love, our health, and the health of our heart. Conversely, loneliness and isolation can be damaging to your health. In addition to surrounding yourself with loving, supportive people, here is a review of the top 10 things you can do from a diet and lifestyle standpoint to help keep your cholesterol in check:

1. *Know your numbers (for blood sugar, blood pressure, and cholesterol)* = proper detection and diagnosis is paramount.
2. *Eat fewer high-cholesterol foods* = especially eggs, meat, shellfish, and dairy
3. *Eat more low-cholesterol foods* = start your day with oatmeal and walnuts, and eat more fish.
4. *Focus on fruits and vegetables* = get five servings every day.
5. *Emphasize essential fatty acids* = avoid saturated and trans fats.

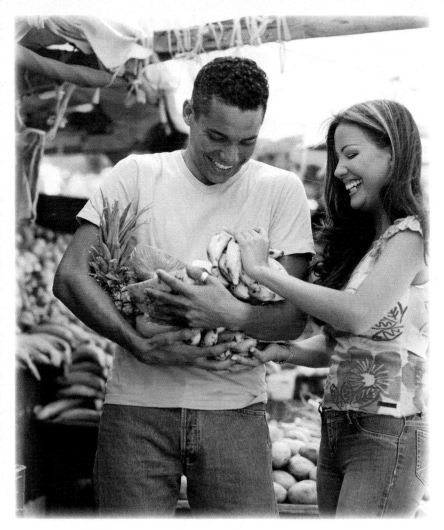

6. **Be physical** = take the stairs, park farther away, and do whatever it takes to become more physically active.

7. **Decrease sodium and increase fiber** = you should eat less than 2,300 mg of sodium a day and at least 20 to 30 grams of fiber.

8. **Stay hydrated** = drink more water and less alcohol and caffeine.

9. **Do not smoke** = also, avoid secondhand smoke whenever possible.

10. **Relax** = make stress reduction a part of your daily routine.

The cholesterol-management goal with diet and lifestyle is to delay or halt the progression of plaque buildup in the arteries or reverse the plaque buildup process entirely. In some cases, dietary supplements should be used to achieve this goal.

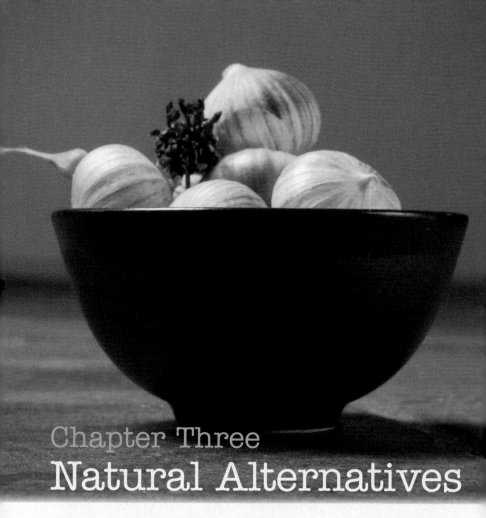

Chapter Three
Natural Alternatives

As a conventionally trained medical doctor, I understand and appreciate the value of strong science. One of the myths associated with "natural medicine" is that these natural substances are not validated using trusted scientific methods. This is true in some cases and not true in others. In the case of cholesterol management—both preventing high cholesterol and lowering elevated levels—there are some natural substances that have proven to be critical tools we can use. In this chapter, I describe some of the natural alternatives that I feel stand up to strong scientific scrutiny.

I have spent the past 15 years researching electron beam CT and multi-detector CT to identify patients at high risk of heart disease. In addition, it is a key research goal of mine to help those patients who discover their high-risk status. For this reason, I have also focused a great deal of attention on studying the effects of aged garlic extract.

Aged Garlic Extract

There are several different types of garlic including raw garlic, garlic oil, crude garlic powders in tablets or capsules, and aged garlic extract as a dietary supplement. I have found that only aged garlic extract provides the concentration and standardization required for effectiveness. In my research, I use the Kyolic brand of aged garlic extract.

Kyolic features garlic that goes through an extensive two-year proprietary aging process that removes the odor-causing compounds and enhances and concentrates the active beneficial components of garlic. I have found that patients and research participants prefer a garlic supplement that is truly odorless. This increases compliance and ensures the product is taken consistently. I also like the fact that Kyolic uses organically grown garlic. Amazingly, there are presently well over 600 published scientific studies in peer-reviewed scientific journals featuring aged garlic extract.

Clinical studies have also shown aged garlic extract is more bioavailable. This means it is found in blood, urine, and body tissue after consumption. Because it is more bioavailable, the body can utilize it more effectively. The aging process also increases the potency of S-allylcysteine (SAC), an important sulfur-containing amino acid. There are only small amounts of SAC in raw garlic. I choose aged garlic for my research because the aging process increases the health benefits of garlic.

I recently presented my most recent research on aged garlic extract at the Experimental Biology 2008 conference and also at two different meetings of the American Heart Association. My colleagues at the Los Angeles Biomedical Research Institute at Harbor-UCLA Medical Center and I demonstrated that aged garlic extract enhances blood flow, clearing arteries of deposits and reducing multiple risk factors for heart disease. In two successive randomized trials, we have shown conclusively that aged garlic extract has cardiovascular benefit.

In one of our studies, we chose to evaluate 65 patients who were at intermediate risk of developing heart disease. We used Kyolic Formula 108 Total Heart Health because in addition to the aged garlic extract, it contains the three key B vitamins (B6, B12, and folate) and L-arginine, a heart-healthy amino acid. The group that took the Kyolic 108 had less calcified plaque progression, lower total cholesterol, and reduced homocysteine levels compared to the participants who received a placebo (fake pill).

We did another study using this same formula and demonstrated it significantly improved circulation and halted calcified plaque progression in the arteries of patients who did not have heart disease symptoms but did have subclinical fatty deposits in the arteries. Half of the study participants took four capsules of the product daily, while the other half took a placebo. Neither the patients nor those administering the capsules knew who was getting the active ingredients and who was getting the fake pill. This is known as a "placebo-controlled, double-blind, randomized trial," which is considered the "gold standard" of research.

Aged garlic extract has a great safety record. The only key contraindication is with the blood-thinning medication warfarin (Coumadin). Garlic supplements and eating raw garlic can negatively interact with this medication so be sure to consult with your physician before taking garlic. Studies with Kyolic aged garlic extract, however, have demonstrated that it is safe to take with prescription anticoagulant medications such as Coumadin. Because garlic can thin the blood, if you are taking a garlic supplement, you should tell your physician prior to any surgical procedure. You will most likely be asked to discontinue the supplement until after the surgery.

My research is demonstrating that when aged garlic extract is combined with other heart-healthy ingredients such as fish oils, vitamin E, B vitamins, and others, it can be even more effective. An important combination is aged garlic extract and CoQ10.

Coenzyme Q10

As mentioned previously, cholesterol-lowering prescription medications can cause a deficiency of CoQ10. This is the most important coenzyme discovered thus far. As a coenzyme, CoQ10 supports energy production on a cellular level. CoQ10 is responsible for transporting an electrical charge across cell membranes. Without this charge, our heart stops pumping, and the brain, liver, kidneys, and other major organs shut down. This consistent energy also helps the body pump out waste, repair damaged tissue, and detoxify.

Foods high in CoQ10 include broccoli, spinach, mackerel, and salmon. CoQ10 is predominantly found in meat. However, some studies have shown that vegetarians actually have higher levels of CoQ10. It is believed that plant foods help protect CoQ10 levels in the body and may even enhance the CoQ10 synthesis that naturally occurs in the body.

In most cases, diet alone will not correct CoQ10 deficiencies. Individuals with heart issues such as high blood pressure, mitral valve prolapse, congestive heart failure, and high cholesterol are at risk of CoQ10 deficiency and may need to supplement the diet. Kyolic Formula 110 provides 300 mg of aged garlic extract with 30 mg of CoQ10. I recommend a minimum of one capsule three times a day.

Editor's Note: For more information about CoQ10, refer to the Coenzyme Q10 Healthy Living Guide by Sherry Torkos, BSc Phm, available at your local, independent health food store.

In addition to aged garlic extract, essential fatty acids such as fish oils, and CoQ10, the research involving plant sterols and heart health, specifically its cholesterol-lowering ability, is impressive.

Plant Sterols

One of the reasons doctors recommend that their patients with high cholesterol increase their consumption of vegetables is because plants contain important compounds called sterols or stanols. These compounds are so important that some manufacturers are fortifying foods with plant sterols and stanols. I prefer a dietary supplement that contains these compounds because it is easier to control the dosage and quality of the product. The makers of ModuCare for immune enhancement have now created Modu-Chol for the successful management of high cholesterol.

Based on a variety of successful clinical studies, the FDA has approved the cholesterol-lowering health claim for plant sterols.

The plant sterols in ModuChol have been proven to help reduce harmful LDL cholesterol levels. The capsules contain a liquid form of these plant sterol compounds for more effective absorption.

Based on a variety of successful clinical studies, the FDA has approved the cholesterol-lowering health claim for plant sterols. In 2007, researchers at East Tennessee State University confirmed the effectiveness of plant sterols. Their study featured 16 participants who took a plant sterol capsule product for four weeks. LDL levels were significantly decreased while HDL levels were increased. Of course, this is the goal of cholesterol medication. These researchers also confirmed the optimum dosage of 1.3 grams per day. Taking two capsules daily of the ModuChol supplies this optimum dosage. Plant sterols should be taken with meals as a part of a diet low in saturated fat and cholesterol.

According to a report in the *Journal of The American College of Nutrition*, South African researchers studied six different published clinical trials and found that plant sterols reduced total cholesterol in people with a family history of high cholesterol. The researchers concluded that plant sterols and stanols offer an effective cholesterol-lowering strategy in this high-risk group.

Plant sterols as a dietary supplement are very safe. However, if you are pregnant or nursing, do not use this supplement without first consulting with your physician. There are no known contraindications or interactions with other supplements or prescription drugs. Some studies have demonstrated that individuals taking statin drugs may have an even greater reduction of LDL cholesterol levels when they add plant sterols. Consistently, the studies have shown that plant sterols can reduce LDL cholesterol by 6 to 15 percent. I recommend ModuChol for people who have been diagnosed with high cholesterol or those with a family history of heart disease or high cholesterol.

Sytrinol

As mentioned previously, cholesterol is manufactured in the liver. The amount of cholesterol that the liver produces can be significant and can also contribute to elevated levels. Several studies have shown that flavonoids found in certain citrus fruits help support effective cholesterol production in the liver. These flavonoids are known in the scientific literature as citrus polymethoxylated flavones. The brand of flavones that has received the most scientific attention is Sytrinol. Preliminary research shows that Sytrinol lowers both cholesterol and triglyceride levels.

A 12-week clinical trial completed recently demonstrated that participants with moderately elevated cholesterol levels who took Sytrinol experienced a 30 percent drop in total cholesterol, 27 percent in LDL cholesterol, and a 34 percent reduction in triglycerides. Sytrinol worked independently of dietary changes. The dosage of Sytrinol is 300 mg per day. Sytrinol is an ingredient in a variety of heart-healthy supplements available at your local natural health store.

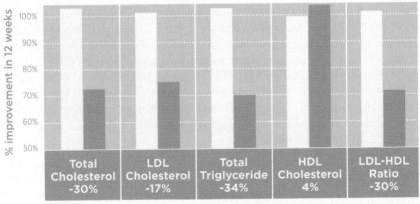

White bars represent subjects consuming placebo for 12 weeks
Blue bars represent subjects consuming Sytrinol™ for 12 weeks

Supplementing The Diet

Dietary supplements are appropriately named because they are meant to be a supplement to a healthy diet. They are not meant to replace healthful eating habits. When combined with a heart-healthy diet, these supplements are even more effective.

In today's fast-paced world, it can be difficult to have a meticulously healthy diet. Food processing, nutrient-deplete soil, and eating on the run can make it hard for us to get all of the heart-healthy nutrients we need from diet alone. That's when the nutrients previously mentioned come in handy.

There are lots of dietary supplements presently available. Yes, nutritional supplements have become big business. That can make it difficult to choose the best supplement for your particular situation. For cholesterol control, I prioritize my recommendations this way (in order of importance):

- Aged garlic extract
- Plant sterols
- CoQ10
- Fish oils
- Sytrinol
- Other supplements such as hawthorn berry, cayenne pepper, and lecithin

It's best to use a supplement that contains as many of the previously listed ingredients as possible. The most important aspect of the nutrients I've listed is that they are scientifically validated and proven to enhance heart health.

Do You Need Supplements?

Dietary supplements are meant to fortify the diet. Here are some key reasons why you may want to consider taking dietary supplements:

- Overprocessing of foods has depleted important nutrients.
- Preservatives, additives, hormones, and artificial flavors and colors contained in nonorganic foods can rob your system of valuable nutrients.
- Smoking, alcohol abuse, and other negative lifestyle factors deplete nutrients.
- Illnesses such as depression, diabetes, and high cholesterol can weaken the body's systems.
- Some prescription drugs can deplete key nutrients.
- Some individuals, such as the elderly, menopausal women, or people with a family history of heart disease, may need additional nutrients.

Chapter Four
Final Thoughts

B y the time you finish reading these last few paragraphs, another person has died of heart disease. Heart disease remains the No. 1 disease killer among North Americans. An estimated 1.2 million Americans will have a new or recurrent heart attack this year (2008 figures from the AHA). As a cardiovascular researcher, I am troubled to know that nearly 50 percent of the time, a deadly heart attack occurs before emergency services or transport to a hospital can even take place. To ease the physical, emotional, and financial burden of this devastating disease, we need to look at reducing risk factors. High cholesterol is a key risk factor for developing heart disease.

In this booklet, I have outlined a comprehensive approach that utilizes early detection, diet, lifestyle, and dietary supplements to help manage healthy cholesterol levels. By using this proactive approach, it may be possible to avoid prescription drugs that have side effects while safely reducing elevated cholesterol and homocysteine levels.

It is critical that you work closely with your doctor. Although many cardiologists or general practitioners may not necessarily be inclined to utilize a more natural approach, it is still important to talk openly with your doctor about your desire to do so. Be sure to inform your doctor about everything you are taking, including all nutritional supplements.

If we are to reduce the number of deaths due to heart disease, we must first address reducing individual risk factors. In large part, heart disease is preventable, and existing heart problems, including high cholesterol, can be reversed. My hope is that the information in this booklet helps you and those you love avoid a heart attack and live a long and vital life.

Selected References

Acuff RV, et al. The lipid lowering effect of plant sterol ester capsules in hypercholesterolemic subjects. *Lipids Health* Dis 6:11, Apr 2007.

Agatston, Arthur. *The South Beach Diet* (St. Martin's Press 2005).

Budoff MJ, et al. Aged garlic extract improves vascular function in asymptomatic individuals with subclinical atherosclerosis. Presented at the Experimental Biology 2008 conference held in San Diego, CA, April 2008.

Budoff MJ, et al. Assessment of coronary artery disease by cardiac computed tomography, a scientific statement from the American Heart Association Committee on Cardiovascular Imaging and Intervention, Council on Cardiovascular Radiology and Intervention, and Committee on Cardiac Imaging, Council on Clinical Cardiology. *Circulation* 114(16):1761-91, 2006.

Budoff MJ, et al. Garlic therapy retards coronary artery calcification. Presented at the Experimental Biology 2008 conference held in San Diego, CA, April 2008.

Budoff MJ, et al. Inhibiting progression of coronary calcification using aged garlic extract in patients receiving statin therapy: a preliminary study. *Prev Med* 39(5):985-91, Nov 2004.

Fu CH, et al. Alterations of cardiovascular autonomic functions by vegetarian diets in postmenopausal women is related to LDL cholesterol levels. Chin J *Physiol* 51(2):100-5, Apr 2008.

Henkin Y, Shai I. Dietary treatment of hypercholesterolemia: Can we predict long-term success? *J Am Coll Nutr* 22(6):555-561, 2003.

Kurowska EM, Manthey JA. Hypolipidemic effects and absorption of citrus polymethoxylated flavones in hamsters with diet-induced hypercholesterolemia. *J Agric Food Chem* 52(10):2879-86, May 2004.

Langsjoen, PH, et al. Treatment of statin adverse effects with supplemental coenzyme Q10 and statin drug discontinuation. *Biofactors* 25(1-4):147-52, 2005.

Li RW, et al. Citrus polymehtoxylated flavones improve lipid and glucose homeostasis and modulate adipocytokines in fructose-induced insulin resistant hamsters. *Life Sci* 79(4):365-73, June 2006.

Moruisi KG, et al. Phytosterols/stanols lower cholesterol concentrations in familial hypercholesterolemic subjects: a systemic review with meta-anaysis. *J Am Coll Nutr* 25(1):41-8, Feb 2006.

Myers J. Exercise and cardiovascular health. *Circulation* 107:e2-e5, 2003.

Niihara, Y, et al. A double blind, randomized, placebo-controlled study of the safety of using aged garlic extract (Kyolic) for patients on oral anticoagulation (Coumadin) therapy. *FASEB J* 18(6):600-605, April 2004.

Olmedilla-Alonso B, et al. Consumption of restructured meat products with added walnuts has a cholesterol-lowering effect in subjects at high cardiovascular risk: a randomized, crossover, placebo-controlled study. *J Am Coll Nutr* 27(2):342-8, Apr 2008.

Passi S, et al. Statins lower plasma and lymphocyte ubiquinol/ubiquinone without affecting other antioxidants and PUFA. *Biofactors* 18(1-4):113-124, 2003.

Rasouli ML, et al. Plasma homocysteine predicts progression of atherosclerosis. *Atherosclerosis* 181(1):159-65, July 2005.

Rocha PM, et al. Independent and opposite associations of hip and waist circumference with metabolic syndrome components and with inflammatory and atherothrombotic risk factors in overweight and obese women. *Metabolism* 57(10):1315-22, Oct 2008.

Roza JM, Xian-Liu Z, Guthrie J. Effect of citrus flavonoids and tocotrienols on serum cholesterol levels in hypercholesterolemic subjects. *Alternative Therapies* 13(6):44-48, Nov/Dec 2007.

Rundek T, et al. Atorvastatin decreases the coenzyme Q10 level in the blood of patients at risk for cardiovascular disease and stroke. *Arch Neurol* 61(6):889-892, Jun 2004.

Schnyder G, et al. Effect of homocysteine-lowering therapy with folic acid, vitamin B12 and vitamin B6 on clinical outcome after percutaneous coronary intervention: the Swiss Heart study: a randomized controlled trial. *JAMA* 288(8):973-9, Aug 2002.

Yeh YY, Liu L. Cholesterol-lowering effect of garlic extracts and organosulfur compounds: human and animal studies. *J Nutr* 131(3s):989S-93S Mar 2001.

http://www.americanheart.org

http://www.americanheart.org/presenter.jhtml?identifier=4506

http://www.nlm.nih.gov/medlineplus/druginfo/medmaster/a608012.html

For more information about the products recommended in this booklet, please visit:

http://www.calciumscan.com

http://www.kyolic.com

http://www.moducare.com